The Plant-Base
course

An Essential Guide To The Best Way
To Reset & Energize Your Body And
Mind With Easy, Healthy Delicious
Recipe

Jason Canon

TABLE OF CONTENTS

Introduction

Thank you very much for purchasing this cookbook. In this cookbook you will find a plant-based diet, it is a diet based mainly on whole plant foods. It is identical to the normal diet we are already used to, except that it leaves out foods that do not come exclusively from plants.

These recipes have been designed just for you who want to lose weight and regain the energy that only a healthy diet can give, but without sacrificing taste.

There are delicious dishes that will have to be recreated with always fresh ingredients to ensure your body assimilates all the nutrients it needs.

Over time, as well as improving your physical fitness, your spirit and mind will also improve. These are the causes of a healthy and balanced diet like the one I am about to propose to you.

I hope you will enjoy cooking my recipes and that they are always to your delight.

Enjoy.

Breakfast Recipes

Indian-Style Lentil and Potato Hash

Preparation time: 10 minutes

Cooking time: 15 minutes

Servings: 4

Ingredients:

¼ cup Vegetable Broth/water, plus more if needed

1 (10-ounce) russet potato, unpeeled, cut into ¼-inch pieces

1 teaspoon ground cumin

½ teaspoon ground allspice

½ teaspoon ground ginger

½ teaspoon garam masala

½ teaspoon salt or Spicy Umami Blend (optional)

1 (15-ounce) can brown lentils, drained and rinsed

½ cup chopped green onions

½ cup chopped fresh cilantro (optional)

¼ cup chopped peanuts (optional)

Directions:

Warm broth over medium-high heat in a large skillet. Add the potato, cumin, allspice, ginger, garam masala, and salt (if using) and cook, frequently stirring, until the potato is tender, about 10 minutes. Put more broth or water as needed to maintain a very thick sauce consistency.

Add the lentils and stir to combine. Adjust the heat to medium, cover, then cook for 5 minutes more.

Divide the lentil mixture among four bowls. Top each serving with 2 tablespoons of green onions, 2 tablespoons of cilantro, and 1 tablespoon of peanuts, then serve.

Nutrition:

Calories: 148

Fat: 1g

Protein: 8g

Carbs: 29g

Maple Muesli

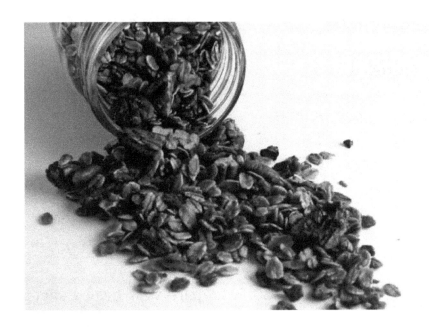

Preparation time: 30 minutes

Cooking time: 20 minutes

Servings: 5

Ingredients:

½ cup dry millet

2 cups rolled oats

1 cup chopped walnuts

½ cup pure maple syrup

1 cup chopped pitted dates

Directions:

Preheat the oven to 350°F. Prepare your baking sheet lined using a parchment paper or a silicone baking mat. Rinse the millet, drain, and shake off as much water as possible. Heat a medium skillet over medium-high heat.

Put the millet in the hot skillet and cook, frequently stirring, until it becomes dry and aromatic and begins to make popping noises, 5 to 8 minutes. Immediately transfer the millet to a large bowl and let cool for 10 minutes.

Add the oats, walnuts, and maple syrup and stir until well combined. Transfer the muesli to the prepared baking sheet and bake for 18 minutes.

Place the baking sheet on a wire rack and let cool. Stir in the dates, then transfer the muesli to an airtight container.

Nutrition:

Calories: 515

Fat: 18g

Protein: 12g

Carbs: 82g

Fruity Yogurt Parfait

Preparation time: 5 minutes

Cooking time: 0 minutes

Servings: 2

Ingredients:

2 cups plain plant-based yogurt or Cashew Cream

2 cups fresh blueberries or raspberries

1 cup Maple Muesli or granola

¼ teaspoon ground cinnamon

Directions:

In an individual serving bowl or parfait glass, layer ½ cup of yogurt, 1 cup of berries, ½ cup of muesli, another ½ cup of yogurt, and 1/8 teaspoon of cinnamon. Repeat in a second serving bowl or parfait glass.

Nutrition:Calories: 520, Fat: 30g, Protein: 14g, Carbs: 71g

Apple Avocado Toast

Preparation time: 5 minutes

Cooking time: 2 minutes

Servings: 4

Ingredients:

1 large ripe avocado, halved and pitted

1 small apple, cored

2 tablespoons lemon juice

½ cup chopped pecans

½ teaspoon ground cinnamon

4 slices whole-grain bread, toasted

Directions:

Scoop your avocado flesh into a small bowl, then mash it with a fork. Cut the apple into 1/8-inch cubes and add it to the avocado.

Add the lemon juice, pecans, and cinnamon and gently fold with a rubber spatula until well combined.

Spread about ¼ cup of the apple-avocado mixture onto each slice of toast and serve.

Nutrition:

Calories: 276

Fat: 19g

Protein: 7g

Carbs: 25g

Lunch Recipes

Green Bean Casserole

Preparation Time: 5 minutes

Cooking Time: 40 minutes

Servings: 4

Ingredients:

6 ounces fried onions

1 ½ cups cremini mushrooms, diced

16 ounces frozen green beans

½ cup diced white onion

1 tablespoon minced garlic

3 ½ tablespoons all-purpose flour

1/3 teaspoon ground black pepper

½ teaspoon dried oregano

3 ½ tablespoons olive oil

2 cups vegetable broth, hot

Directions:

Switch on the oven, then set it to 400 degrees F and let it preheat.

Take a medium saucepan, place it over medium heat, add oil and when hot, add onion and mushrooms, stir in garlic and cook for 4 minutes until tender.

Stir in flour until the thick paste comes together and then cook for 2 minutes until golden.

Stir in vegetable broth, bring it to a simmer, then stir in black pepper and oregano, whisk well and cook for 15 minutes until gravy thickened to the desired level.

Add green beans, stir until mixed, remove the pan from heat, top beans with fried onions and bake for 15 minutes.

Serve straight away.

Nutrition: 191 Cal 10 g Fat 2 g Saturated Fat 22 g Carbohydrates 3.3 g Fiber 2.5 g Sugars 4.1 g Protein;

Pumpkin Risotto

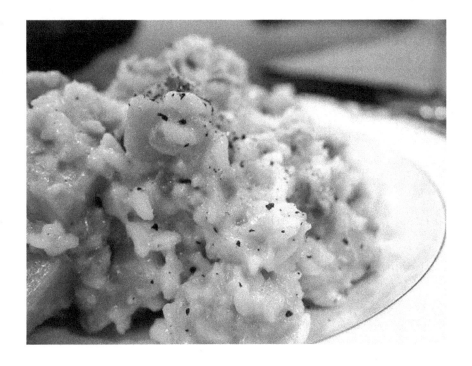

Preparation Time: 5 minutes

Cooking Time: 20 minutes

Servings: 4

Ingredients:

1 cup Arborio rice

½ cup cooked and chopped pumpkin

1/2 cup mushrooms

1 rib of celery, diced

½ of a medium white onion, peeled, diced

½ teaspoon minced garlic

½ teaspoon salt

1/3 teaspoon ground black pepper

1 tablespoon olive oil

½ tablespoon coconut butter

1 cup pumpkin puree

2 cups vegetable stock

Directions:

Take a medium saucepan, place it over medium heat, add oil and when hot, add onion and celery, stir in garlic and cook for 3 minutes until onions begin to soften.

Add mushrooms, season with salt and black pepper and cook for 5 minutes.

Add rice, pour in pumpkin puree, then gradually pour in the stock until rice soaked up all the liquid and have turned soft.

Add butter, remove the pan from heat, stir until creamy mixture comes together, and then serve.

Nutrition: 218.5 Cal 5.2 g Fat 1.5 g Saturated Fat 32.3 g Carbohydrates 1.3 g Fiber 3.8 g Sugars 6.3 g Protein;

Brown Rice and Vegetable Stir-Fry

Preparation Time: 5 minutes

Cooking Time: 50 minutes

Servings: 4

Ingredients:

16-ounce tofu, extra-firm, pressed, drained, cut into ½-inch cubes

1 cup of brown rice

1 cup frozen broccoli florets

1 medium red bell pepper, cored, diced

1 small white onion, peeled, diced

1 tablespoon minced garlic

½ teaspoon salt

1/3 teaspoon ground black pepper

1 tablespoon olive oil

2 cups vegetable broth

Directions:

Take a medium pot, place it over high heat, add brown rice, pour in vegetable broth, and bring it to a boil.

Switch heat to medium-low level, cover the pot with the lid and cook for 40 minutes, and when done, remove the pot and set aside until required.

Then take a large skillet pan, place it over medium-high heat, add oil and when hot, add tofu pieces, onion, broccoli, and bell pepper, season with salt and black pepper and cook for 5 minutes until sauté.

Add cooked rice, stir until mixed and continue cooking for 5 minutes.

Serve straight away.

Nutrition: 281.9 Cal 11.7 g Fat 1.7 g Saturated Fat

31.1 g Carbohydrates 9.7 g Fiber 2.1 g Sugars 20.1 g Protein;

Tomato Basil Spaghetti

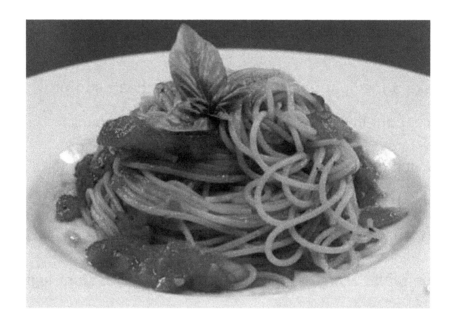

Preparation Time: 5 minutes

Cooking Time: 20 minutes

Servings: 4

Ingredients:

15-ounce cooked great northern beans

10.5-ounces cherry tomatoes, halved

1 small white onion, peeled, diced

1 tablespoon minced garlic

8 basil leaves, chopped

2 tablespoons olive oil

1-pound spaghetti

Directions:

Take a large pot half full with salty water, place it over medium-high heat, bring it to a boil, add spaghetti and cook for 10 to 12 minutes until tender.

Then drain spaghetti into a colander and reserve 1 cup of pasta liquid.

Take a large skillet pan, place it over medium-high heat, add oil and when hot, add onion, tomatoes, basil, and garlic and cook for 5 minutes until vegetables have turned tender.

Add cooked spaghetti and beans, pour in pasta water, stir until just mixed and cook for 2 minutes until hot.

Serve straight away.

Nutrition: 147 Cal 5 g Fat 0.7 g Saturated Fat 21.2 g Carbohydrates 1.5 g Fiber 5.4 g Sugars 3.8 g Protein;

Dinner Recipes

Bean and Carrot Spirals

Preparation Time: 10 minutes

Cooking Time: 40 minutes

Servings: 24

Ingredients:

4 8-inch flour tortillas

1 ½ cups of Easy Mean White Bean dip

10 ounces spinach leaves

½ cup diced carrots

½ cup diced red peppers

Directions:

Starts by preparing the bean dip, seen above. Next, spread out the bean dip on each tortilla, making sure to leave about a ¾ inch white border on the tortillas' surface. Next, place spinach in the center of the tortilla, followed by carrots and red peppers.

Roll the tortillas into tight rolls, and cover every roll with plastic wrap or aluminum foil.

Let them chill in the fridge for twenty-four hours.

Afterward, remove the wrap from the spirals and remove the very ends of the rolls. Slice the rolls into six individual spiral pieces, and arrange them on a platter for serving. Enjoy!

Nutrition:

Calories: 205 kcal

Protein: 6.41 g

Fat: 4.16 g

Carbohydrates: 35.13 g

Tofu Nuggets with Barbecue Glaze

Preparation Time: 10 minutes

Cooking Time: 25 minutes

Servings: 9

Ingredients:

32 ounces tofu

1 cup quick vegan barbecue sauce

Directions:

Set the oven to 425F.

Next, slice the tofu and blot the tofu with clean towels. Next, slice and dice the tofu and completely eliminate the water from the tofu material.

Stir the tofu with the vegan barbecue sauce, and place the tofu on a baking sheet.

Bake the tofu for fifteen minutes. Afterward, stir the tofu and bake the tofu for an additional ten minutes.

Enjoy!

Nutrition: Calories: 311 kcal , Protein: 19.94 g , Fat: 21.02 g , Carbohydrates: 15.55 g

Peppered Pinto Beans

Preparation Time: 10 minutes

Cooking Time: 15 minutes

Servings: 6

Ingredients:

1 tsp. Chili powder

1 tsp. ground cumin

.5 cup Vegetable

2 cans Pinto beans

1 Minced jalapeno

1 Diced red bell pepper

1 tsp. Olive oil

Directions:

Take out a pot and heat the oil. Cook the jalapeno and pepper for a bit before adding in the pepper, salt, cumin, broth, and beans.

Place to a boil and then reduce the heat to cook for a bit. After 10 minutes, let it cool and serve.

Nutrition:

Calories: 183

Carbs: 32g

Fat: 2g

Protein: 11g

Black Bean Pizza

Preparation Time: 30 minutes

Cooking Time: 20 minutes

Servings: 2

Ingredients:

1 Sliced avocado

1 Sliced red onion

1 Grated carrot

1 Sliced tomato

.5 cup Spicy black bean dip

2 Pizza crusts

Directions:

Turn on the oven and let heat to 400 degrees. Layout two crusts on a baking sheet and add the dip onto each one.

Top with the tomato slices and sprinkle the carrots and the onion on a well.

Add to the oven and let it bake for about 20 minutes or so until done. Top with the avocado before serving.

Nutrition:

Calories: 379

Carbs: 59g

Fat: 13g

Protein: 13g

Vegetables Recipes

Quinoa Avocado Salad

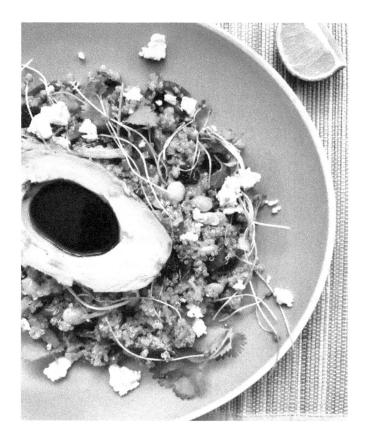

Preparation Time: 15 minutes

Cooking Time: 4 minutes

Servings: 4

Ingredients:

2 tablespoons balsamic vinegar

¼ cup cream

¼ cup buttermilk

5 tablespoons lemon juice

1 clove garlic, grated

2 tablespoons shallot, minced

Salt and pepper to taste

2 tablespoons avocado oil, divided

1 ¼ cups quinoa, cooked

2 heads endive, sliced

2 firm pears, sliced thinly

2 avocados, sliced

¼ cup fresh dill, chopped

Direction

Combine the vinegar, cream, milk, 1 tablespoon lemon juice, garlic, shallot, salt and pepper in a bowl.

Pour 1 tablespoon oil into a pan over medium heat.

Heat the quinoa for 4 minutes.

Transfer quinoa to a plate.

Toss the endive and pears in a mixture of remaining oil, remaining lemon juice, salt and pepper.

Transfer to a plate.

Toss the avocado in the reserved dressing.

Add to the plate.

Top with the dill and quinoa.

Nutrition:

431 Calories

6g Fiber

6.6g Protein

Roasted Sweet Potatoes

Preparation Time: 20 minutes

Cooking Time: 20 minutes

Servings: 4

Ingredients:

2 potatoes, sliced into wedges

2 tablespoons olive oil, divided

Salt and pepper to taste

1 red bell pepper, chopped

¼ cup fresh cilantro, chopped

1 garlic, minced

2 tablespoons almonds, toasted and sliced

1 tablespoon lime juice

Direction

Preheat your oven to 425 degrees F.

Toss the sweet potatoes in oil and salt.

Transfer to a baking pan.

Roast for 20 minutes.

In a bowl, combine the red bell pepper, cilantro, garlic and almonds.

In another bowl, mix the lime juice, remaining oil, salt and pepper.

Drizzle this mixture over the red bell pepper mixture.

Serve sweet potatoes with the red bell pepper mixture.

Nutrition:

146 Calories

2.9g Fiber

2.3g Protein

Garlic Mashed Potatoes & Turnips

Preparation Time: 20 minutes

Cooking Time: 30 minutes

Servings: 8

Ingredients:

1 head garlic

1 teaspoon olive oil

1 lb. turnips, sliced into cubes

2 lb. potatoes, sliced into cubes

½ cup almond milk

½ cup Parmesan cheese, grated

1 tablespoon fresh thyme, chopped

1 tablespoon fresh chives, chopped

2 tablespoons butter

Direction

Preheat your oven to 375 degrees F.

Slice the tip off the garlic head.

Dash little oil and roast in the oven for 45 minutes.

Boil the turnips and potatoes in a pot of water for 30 minutes or until tender.

Incorporate all the ingredients to a food processor along with the garlic.

Pulse until smooth.

Nutrition:

141 Calories

3.1g Fiber

4.6g Protein

Green Beans

Preparation Time: 15 minutes

Cooking Time: 20 minutes

Servings: 8

Ingredients:

1 shallot, chopped

24 oz. green beans

Salt and pepper to taste

½ teaspoon smoked paprika

1 teaspoon lemon juice

2 teaspoons vinegar

Direction

Preheat your oven to 450 degrees F.

Stir in the shallot and beans.

Season with salt, pepper and paprika.

Roast for 10 minutes.

Drizzle with the lemon juice and vinegar.

Roast for another 2 minutes.

Nutrition:

49 Calories

3g Fiber

2.9g Protein

Finger Food

Choco Coffee Energy Shake

Preparation time: 10 minutes

Cooking time: 0 minutes

Servings: 1

Ingredients:

2 scoops of chocolate protein powder

1/2 cup of low-fat milk

1 cup of water

1 tablespoon of instant coffee

Directions:

Add all the Ingredients: to a blender and blend until smooth

Enjoy

Nutrition: Calories per serving: 299 , Protein: 42g , Carbs: 14g , Fat: 6g

Lean and Mean Pineapple Shake

Preparation time: 10 minutes

Cooking time: 0 minutes

Servings: 1

Ingredients:

1 cup chopped fresh pineapple

4 strawberries

1 banana

1 tablespoon low-fat Greek yogurt

1 scoop of vanilla protein powder

1 cup of water

Directions:

Add all the Ingredients: to a blender and blend until smooth.

Enjoy

Nutrition Calories per serving: 355 , Protein: 23g , Carbs: 65g , Fat: 3g

Chopped Almond Smoothie

Preparation time: 10 minutes

Cooking time: 0 minutes

Servings: 1

Ingredients:

1 1/2 cups water

17 chopped almonds

1/2 teaspoon coconut extract

1 scoop chocolate protein powder

Directions:

Add all the Ingredients: to a blender and blend until smooth

Enjoy

Nutrition: Calories per serving: 241 , Protein: 24g , Carbs: 6g , Fat: 13g

Vanilla Strawberry Surprise

Preparation time: 10 minutes

Cooking time: 0 minutes

Servings: 1

Ingredients:

2 scoops of vanilla protein powder

1 cup of ice

1 banana

4 fresh or frozen strawberries

Directions:

Add all the Ingredients: to a blender and blend until smooth.

Enjoy

Nutrition: Calories per serving: 329 , Protein: 36g Carbs: 42g Fat: 2g

Breakfast Banana Shake

Preparation time: 10 minutes

Cooking time: 0 minutes

Servings: 1

Ingredients:

3/4 cup of low-fat milk

1 banana

1/4 pound of rolled oats

2 scoops of vanilla whey protein powder

Directions:

Add all the Ingredients: to a blender and blend until smooth

Enjoy

Nutrition: Calories per serving: 566 , Protein: 59g Carbs: 69g Fat: 6g

Berry Beetsicle Smoothie

Preparation time: 3 minutes

Servings: 1

Ingredients:

1/2 cup peeled and diced beets

1/2 cup frozen raspberries

1 frozen banana

1 tablespoon maple syrup

1 cup unsweetened soy or almond milk

Directions:

Combine all the Ingredients: in a blender and blend until smooth.

Nutrition:

Calories: 130, Protein 9 g, Fat 3 g,

Carbs 28 g, Fiber 11 g

Green Breakfast Smoothie

Preparation time: 10 minutes

Servings: 2

Ingredients:

1/2 banana, sliced

2 cups spinach or other greens, such as kale

1 cup sliced berries of your choosing, fresh or frozen

1 orange, peeled and cut into segments

1 cup unsweetened non-dairy milk

1 cup ice

Directions:

In a blender, combine all the Ingredients:

Starting with the blender on low speed, begin blending the smoothie, gradually increasing blender speed until smooth.

Serve immediately.

Nutrition: Calories: 100, Protein 4 g, Fat 3 g, Carbs 20 g, Fiber 10 g

Blueberry Lemonade Smoothie

Preparation time: 5 minutes

Servings: 1

Ingredients:

1 cup roughly chopped kale

3/4 cup frozen blueberries

1 cup unsweetened soy or almond milk

Juice of 1 lemon

1 tablespoon maple syrup

Directions:

Combine all the Ingredients: in a blender and blend until smooth. Serve immediately.

Nutrition:

Calories: 95, Protein 5 g, Fat 6 g, Carbs 22 g, Fiber 11 g

Berry Protein Smoothie

Preparation time: 5 minutes

Servings: 1

Ingredients:

1 banana

1 cup fresh or frozen berries

3/4 cup water or nondairy milk, plus more as needed

1 scoop plant-based protein powder

3 ounces silken tofu

1/4 cup rolled oats, or ½ cup cooked quinoa

Additions

1 tablespoon ground flaxseed or chia seeds

1 handful fresh spinach or lettuce, or 1 chunk cucumber

Coconut water to replace some of the liquid

Directions:

In a blender, combine the banana, berries, water, and your choice of protein. Add any addition Ingredients: as desired. Purée until smooth and creamy, about 50 seconds.

Add a bit more water if you like a thinner smoothie.

Nutrition:

Calories: 180,

Protein 18 g,

Fat 5 g,

Carbs 30 g,

Fiber 11 g

Soup and Stew

Avocado Mint Soup

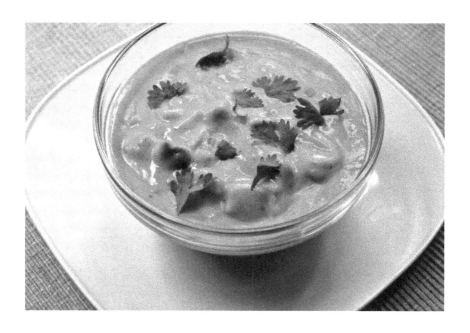

Preparation Time: 10 minutes

Cooking Time: 10 minutes

Servings: 2

Ingredients:

1 medium avocado, peeled, pitted, and cut into pieces

1 cup coconut milk

2 romaine lettuce leaves

20 fresh mint leaves

1 tbsp fresh lime juice

1/8 tsp salt

Directions:

Add all ingredients into the blender and blend until smooth. Soup should be thick not as a puree.

Pour into the serving bowls and place in the refrigerator for 10 minutes.

Stir well and serve chilled.

Nutrition: Calories: 377 kcal, Fat: 14.9g , Carbs: 60.7g , Protein: 6.4g

Creamy Squash Soup

Preparation Time: 10 minutes

Cooking Time: 25 minutes

Servings: 8

Ingredients:

3 cups butternut squash, chopped

1 ½ cups unsweetened coconut milk

1 tbsp coconut oil

1 tsp dried onion flakes

1 tbsp curry powder

4 cups water

1 garlic clove

1 tsp kosher salt

Directions:

Add squash, coconut oil, onion flakes, curry powder, water, garlic, and salt into a large saucepan. Bring to boil over high heat.

Turn heat to medium and simmer for 20 minutes.

Puree the soup using a blender until smooth. Return soup to the saucepan and stir in coconut milk and cook for 2 minutes.

Stir well and serve hot.

Nutrition:

Calories: 271 kcal

Fat: 3.7g

Carbs: 54g

Protein:6.5g

Zucchini Soup

Preparation Time: 10 minutes

Cooking Time: 15 minutes

Servings: 8

Ingredients:

2 ½ lbs. zucchini, peeled and sliced

1/3 cup basil leaves

4 cups vegetable stock

4 garlic cloves, chopped

2 tbsp olive oil

1 medium onion, diced

Pepper

Salt

Directions:

Heat olive oil in a pan over medium-low heat.

Add zucchini and onion and sauté until softened. Add garlic and sauté for a minute.

Add vegetable stock and simmer for 15 minutes.

Remove from heat. Stir in basil and puree the soup using a blender until smooth and creamy. Season with pepper and salt.

Stir well and serve.

Nutrition:

Calories: 434 kcal

Fat: 35g

Carbs: 27g

Protein: 6.7g

Appetizer

Jicama and Guacamole

Preparation time: 15 minutes

Cooking time: 0 minutes

Servings: 4

Ingredients:

juice of 1 lime, or 1 tablespoon prepared lime juice

2 hass avocados, peeled, pits removed, and cut into cubes

½ teaspoon sea salt

½ red onion, minced

1 garlic clove, minced

¼ cup chopped cilantro (optional)

1 jicama bulb, peeled and cut into matchsticks

Directions:

In a medium bowl, squeeze the lime juice over the top of the avocado and sprinkle with salt. Lightly mash the avocado with a fork. Stir in the onion, garlic, and cilantro, if using.

Serve with slices of jicama to dip in guacamole. To store, place plastic wrap over the bowl of guacamole and refrigerate. The guacamole will keep for about 2 days.

Nutrition:

Calories: 145

Carbs: 0g

Fat: 10g

Protein: 9g

Tempeh Tantrum Burgers

Preparation time: 15 minutes

Cooking time: 14 minutes

Servings: 4

Ingredients:

8 ounces tempeh, cut into ½-inch dice

¾ cup chopped onion

2 garlic cloves, chopped

¾ cup chopped walnuts

½ cup old-fashioned or quick-cooking oats

1 tablespoon minced fresh parsley

½ teaspoon dried oregano

½ teaspoon dried thyme

½ teaspoon salt

¼ teaspoon freshly ground black pepper

3 tablespoons extra-virgin olive oil

Dijon mustard

4 whole grain burger rolls

Sliced red onion, tomato, lettuce, and avocado

Directions:

Cook the tempeh within 30 minutes in a medium saucepan of simmering water. Drain and set aside to cool.

Combine the onion and garlic in a food processor then process until minced. Put the cooled tempeh, the walnuts, oats, parsley, oregano, thyme, salt, and pepper. Process until well blended. Shape the mixture into 4 equal patties.

Heat-up the oil in a large skillet on medium heat. Add the burgers and cook until cooked thoroughly and browned on both sides for about 7 minutes per side.

Spread desired amount of mustard onto each half of the rolls and layer each roll with lettuce, tomato, red onion, and avocado as desired. Serve immediately.

Nutrition:

Calories: 150

Carbs: 8g

Fat: 7g

Protein: 13g

Sesame- Wonton Crisps

Preparation time: 15 minutes

Cooking time: 10 minutes

Servings: 12

Ingredients:

12 Vegan Wonton Wrappers

2 tablespoons toasted sesame oil

12 shiitake mushrooms, lightly rinsed, patted dry, stemmed, and cut into 1/4-inch slices

4 snow peas, trimmed and cut crosswise into thin slivers

1 teaspoon soy sauce

1 tablespoon fresh lime juice

½ teaspoon brown sugar

1 medium carrot, shredded

Toasted sesame seeds or black sesame seeds, if available

Directions:

Preheat the oven to 350°F. Oil a baking sheet and set aside. Brush the wonton wrappers with 1 tablespoon of the sesame oil and arrange on the baking sheet.

Bake until golden brown and crisp within 5 minutes. Set aside to cool. (Alternately, you can tuck the wonton wrappers into mini-muffin tins to create cups for the filling. Brush with sesame oil and bake them until crisp.)

In a large skillet, heat the extra olive oil over medium heat. Add the mushrooms and cook until softened. Stir in the snow peas and the soy sauce and cook for 30 seconds. Set aside to cool.

In a large bowl, combine the lime juice, sugar, and remaining 1 tablespoon sesame oil. Stir in the carrot and cooled shiitake mixture.

Top each wonton crisp with a spoonful of the shiitake mixture. Sprinkle with sesame seeds and arrange on a platter to serve.

Nutrition:

Calories: 88

Carbs: 14g

Fat: 2g

Protein: 3g

Macadamia-Cashew Patties

Preparation time: 15 minutes

Cooking time: 10 minutes

Servings: 4

Ingredients:

¾ cup chopped macadamia nuts

¾ cup chopped cashews

1 medium carrot, grated

1 small onion, chopped

1 garlic clove, minced

1 jalapeño or another green chili, seeded and minced

¾ cup old-fashioned oats

¾ cup dry unseasoned bread crumbs

2 tablespoons minced fresh cilantro

½ teaspoon ground coriander

Salt and freshly ground black pepper

2 teaspoons fresh lime juice

Canola or grapeseed oil, for frying

4 sandwich rolls

Lettuce leaves and condiment of choice

Directions:

In a food processor, combine the macadamia nuts, cashews, carrot, onion, garlic, chili, oats, bread crumbs, cilantro, coriander, and salt and pepper.

Process until well mixed. Add the lime juice and process until well blended. Taste, adjusting the seasonings if necessary. Shape the mixture into 4 equal patties.

Heat-up a thin layer of oil in a large skillet over medium heat. Add the patties and cook until golden brown on both sides, turning once, for about 10 minutes in total.

Serve on sandwich rolls with lettuce and condiments of choice.

Nutrition:

Calories: 190

Carbs: 7g

Fat: 17g

Protein: 4g

Drinks

Chocolate and Cherry Smoothie

Preparation Time: 5 minutes

Cooking Time: 0 minute

Servings: 2

Ingredients:

4 cups frozen cherries

2 tablespoons cocoa powder

1 scoop of protein powder

1 teaspoon maple syrup

2 cups almond milk, unsweetened

Directions:

1.   Place all the ingredients in the order in a food processor or blender and then pulse for 2 to 3 minutes at high speed until smooth.

2.   Pour the smoothie into two glasses and then serve.

Nutrition: Calories: 247 Fat: 3g Protein: 18g Sugar: 3g

Strawberry Shake

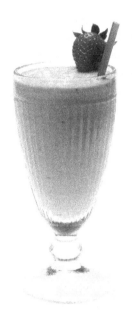

Preparation Time: 10 minutes

Cooking Time: 10 minutes

Servings: 2

Ingredients:

1½ cups fresh strawberries, hulled

1 large frozen banana, peeled

2 scoops unsweetened vegan vanilla protein powder

2 tablespoons hemp seeds

2 cups unsweetened hemp milk

Directions:

In a high-speed blender, place all the ingredients and pulse until creamy.

Pour into two glasses and serve immediately.

Nutrition: Calories: 259 Fat: 3g Protein: 10g Sugar: 2g

Chocolatey Banana Shake

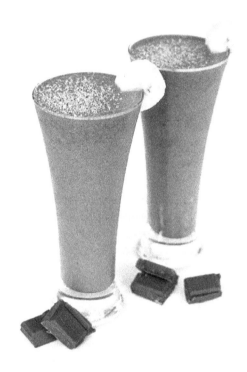

Preparation Time: 10 minutes

Cooking Time: 10 minutes

Servings: 2

Ingredients:

2 medium frozen bananas, peeled

4 dates, pitted

4 tablespoons peanut butter

4 tablespoons rolled oats

2 tablespoons cacao powder

2 tablespoons chia seeds

2 cups unsweetened soymilk

Directions:

Place all the ingredients in a high-speed blender and pulse until creamy.

Pour into two glasses and serve immediately.

Nutrition: Calories: 502 Fat: 4g Protein: 11g Sugar: 9g

Fruity Tofu Smoothie

Preparation Time: 10 minutes

Cooking Time: 10 minutes

Servings: 2

Ingredients:

12 ounces silken tofu, pressed and drained

2 medium bananas, peeled

1½ cups fresh blueberries

1 tablespoon maple syrup

1½ cups unsweetened soymilk

¼ cup ice cubes

Directions:

Place all the ingredients in a high-speed blender and pulse until creamy.

Pour into two glasses and serve immediately.

Nutrition: Calories 235 Carbohydrates: 1.9g Protein: 14.3g Fat: 18.9g

Dessert Recipes

Chocomint Hazelnut Bars

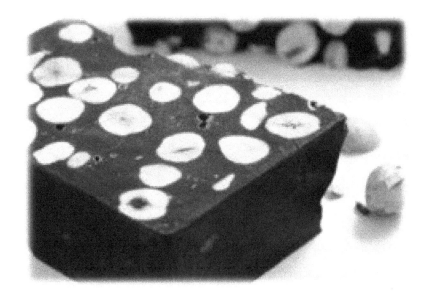

Preparation Time: 5 minutes

Cooking Time: 15 minutes

Servings: 8

Ingredients:

1/2 cup coconut oil, melted

4 Tbsp cocoa powder

1/4 cup almond butter

3/4 cup brown sugar - (packed)

1 tsp vanilla extract

1 tsp pure peppermint extract

pinch of salt

1 cup shredded coconut

1 cup hazelnuts sliced

Directions:

Chop the hazelnuts in a food processor; set aside.

Fill the bottom of a double boiler with water and place it on low heat.

Put the coconut oil, cacao powder, almond butter, brown sugar, vanilla, peppermint extract, and salt in the top of a double boiler over hot (not boiling) water and constantly stir for 10 minutes.

Add hazelnuts and shredded coconut to the melted mixture and stir together.

Pour the mixture in a dish lined with parchment and freeze for several hours.

Remove from the freezer and cut into bars.

Store in airtight container or freezer bag in a freezer.

Let the bars at room temperature for 10 to 15 minutes before eating.

Nutrition: Calories: 186 Total Fat: 4g Saturated Fat: 0g Cholesterol: 33mg Sodium: 783mg Carbohydrates: 23g Fiber: 6g Protein: 19g

Coco-Cinnamon Balls

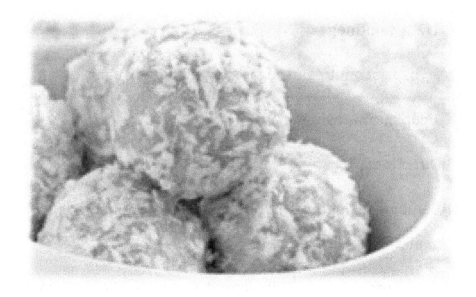

Preparation Time: 10 minutes

Cooking Time: 5 minutes

Servings: 12

Ingredients:

1 cup coconut butter softened

1 cup coconut milk canned

1 tsp pure vanilla extract

3/4 tsp cinnamon

1/2 tsp nutmeg

2 Tbsp coconut palm sugar (or granulated sugar)

1 cup coconut shreds

Directions:

Combine all ingredients (except the coconut shreds) in a heated bath - bain-marie.

Cook and stir until all ingredients are soft and well combined.

Remove bowl from heat, place into a bowl, and refrigerate until the mixture firmed up.

Form cold coconut mixture into balls, and roll each ball in the shredded coconut.

Store into a sealed container, and keep refrigerated up to one week.

Nutrition: Calories: 213 Fat: 6g Fiber: 13g Carbs: 16g Protein: 22g

Chocolate and Avocado Pudding

Preparation Time: 3 hours and 10 minutes

Cooking Time: 0 minute

Servings: 1

Ingredients:

1 small avocado, pitted, peeled

1 small banana, mashed

1/3 cup cocoa powder, unsweetened

1 tablespoon cacao nibs, unsweetened

1/4 cup maple syrup

1/3 cup coconut cream

Directions:

Add avocado in a food processor along with cream and then pulse for 2 minutes until smooth.

Add remaining ingredients, blend until mixed, and then tip the pudding in a container.

Cover the container with a plastic wrap; it should touch the pudding and refrigerate for 3 hours.

Serve straight away.

Nutrition: Calories: 87 Cal Fat: 7 g Carbs: 9 g Protein: 1.5 g Fiber: 3.2 g

Chocolate Avocado Ice Cream

Preparation Time: 1 hour and 10 minutes

Cooking Time: 0 minute

Servings: 2

Ingredients:

4.5 ounces avocado, peeled, pitted

1/2 cup cocoa powder, unsweetened

1 tablespoon vanilla extract, unsweetened

1/2 cup and 2 tablespoons maple syrup

13.5 ounces coconut milk, unsweetened

1/2 cup water

Directions:

Add avocado in a food processor along with milk and then pulse for 2 minutes until smooth.

Add remaining ingredients, blend until mixed, and then tip the pudding in a freezer-proof container.

Place the container in a freezer and chill for freeze for 4 hours until firm, whisking every 20 minutes after 1 hour.

Serve straight away.

Nutrition: Calories: 80.7 Cal Fat: 7.1 g Carbs: 6 g Protein: 0.6 g Fiber: 2 g

Conclusion

Congratulations on making it to the end of this cookbook. The plant-based diet has several positive characteristics, it's easy to follow, and the meals are delicious, not like everyone is trying to tell you. In addition, it will bring you many benefits, such as weight loss and better health.

Without commitment, however, it will be impossible for you to achieve the goals set. Develop a practical plan that will help you transition smoothly to the plant-based lifestyle and you will see that your journey will be simple and effective.

Good luck!